GLUTEN FREE AND HEALTHY DESSERTS

Joan D. Phillips

Copyright © 2022 by Joan D. Phillips

All rights reserved.

No portion of this book may be reproduced in any form without written permission from the publisher or author, except as permitted by U.S. copyright law.

Contents

Chapter One

INTRODUCTION

To all the foodies and dessert lovers out there—those who want to savour only the purest of sweets while still feeling good about it—this book is devoted. My goal is to provide novel, tasty, and nutritious options for making desserts including cakes, cookies, ice cream, and other sweets.

When it comes to savouring a dessert, I believe true enjoyment implies that you still feel fantastic, fresh, and guilt-free after you've eaten it. So I've swapped out low-quality ingredients for fresh and healthful ones. Ingredients that could make you sick have been omitted from my recipes in favour of those that would lift your spirits. Sweets don't have to be vices; they may be virtues, too!

Natural flavours and wholesome raw ingredients are respected in my dishes, while white sugar and wheat are joyfully ignored. You may end up feeling worse as a result of these products. And they're unnecessary. When it comes to baking, there are better options for both of these.

My recipes are built around fresh, whole foods that haven't been tampered with in any way. I want to make desserts that are simple to make, but yet appealing to those with more baking experience. No heating is required in half the recipes in this book to maintain the quality of its ingredients. Gluten, dairy, and yeast-free dishes are included in the book. So that all people can locate and create their own favourite sweets, many of the recipes are grain-free and vegan, or can be created without animal products.

All of the recipes and photographs on this site were created by me. Everything on this menu has been made with care, and I've personally taste-tested every item. Please remember to treat your body with respect, eat only the greatest food, and enjoy sweets guilt-free with my book!

Become a modern-day dessert foodie and give in to your cravings!

CONTENT DETAILED

You can find everything you need at a grocery store or health food store, or you can order it online from a number of different sources. They can be created at home in some situations.

Extracts and Flour

Flour made of almonds. One of my favourites is this high-fiber, flavorful flour. A lack of structure in the dough is a problem for almond flour, as well as many gluten-free flours. Baking powder and psyllium powder will work together to form a binding agent. Raw almonds can also be used to make coarser almond meal. Because it includes more oil, coarse almond meal tends to be less absorbent than finely ground almond flour.

FLOUR FROM COCONUT. My second favourite is coconut flour that is naturally sweetened. It can be used with or substituted for almond flour. Coconut flour absorbs liquid from other ingredients, so you often only need one-third the amount of conventional flour in most recipes.

NUT FLOUR. Nut flours can be used for any flour to create unique flavours. Seed flours, such as pumpkin seed flour, can be used by those who are sensitive to nuts. You may grind your own nut flour by using a high-speed blender to process the nuts. The flour should not be over-ground in order to avoid converting into nut butter, which can be used in baking as well.

Oatmeal Flour. A high-speed blender can be used to ground gluten-free oats into gluten-free oat flour at home. Oat flour provides excellent structure, but it can quickly transform the dough into a paste. Xanthan gum or psyllium husk powder can be added to the mix.

POWDER OF PSYLLIUM HUSK. Plantain seeds are used to make this powder, which absorbs water. In gluten-free baking, it provides structure and fluffiness. It also makes it easier to handle dough.

FLOUR OF TAPIOCA. Cassava, a tropical root, is used to make the mild-tasting tapioca flour. Pastries can benefit from the addition of moisture and texture, or they can be thickened with it.

This product contains XANTHAN GUM. Sugar is fermented in a liquid to create this powder, which lends a textured and dimensional quality. When making cakes and cookies, it's better to combine it with flour.

Flour with Chia Seeds. When mixed with water, flaxseeds and chia seeds form a gel. In baking, the gel can be employed to add structure. A spice grinder or a flaxseed mill can be used to grind the seeds to a fine powder. Mix 3 tablespoons of water with 1 tablespoon of ground flaxseeds. For 15 minutes, put the mixture in the fridge. A "flaxseed egg" can be substituted for eggs in many recipes.

COOKIES WITH ANISE AND FIGS

Allow me to introduce one of my favourite cookies! When anise and fig are combined, the result is a delicious licorice flavour. The flavour is enhanced by a coating of licorice powder. These cookies are made much better with a hint of almond.

MAKES APPROXIMATELY 16 COOKIES

1 cup flour made from buckwheat

12 CUP ALMONDFILLER

12 CUP COCONUT SUCTION

14 cup flaxseed, ground

1 tablespoon star anise powder

1 teaspoon powdered baking soda

a quarter teaspoon of salt

12 cup oat milk (or other milk substitute) (see recipe)

14 cup melted coconut oil and/or butter

1 teaspoon extract de vanille

12 cup almonds, flaked

7 dried figs, peeled and cut into little pieces

As required, rehydrate

ABOVE ALL

powdered licorice

In a mixing bowl, combine the flours, coconut sugar, flaxseed, star anise, baking powder, and sea salt. Combine the oat milk, coconut oil, and vanilla essence in a separate bowl. Combine the wet and dry ingredients in a mixing bowl. Combine the almonds and figs in a mixing bowl. The dough should be firm, pliable, and easy to work with. If required, add some water.

Roll the dough into a log about 2 inches in diameter. Refrigerate for 30 minutes or freeze for 15 minutes after wrapping in plastic wrap.

Preheat the oven to 350 degrees Fahrenheit and prepare a baking sheet with parchment paper. Remove the plastic wrap from the dough log and let it to cool to room temperature. Using a 12-inch slicer, cut the log into 12-inch pieces. Place the pieces on the baking sheet that has been prepared. Add a pinch of licorice powder to each one. Preheat oven to 350°F and bake for 10 minutes. Bake for another 10 minutes after carefully flipping the cookies. Allow to cool completely before serving. Serve and have fun!

COOKIES WITH LACE

These lovely paper-thin lace cookies come together quickly. They'll appeal to anyone who enjoys Swedish Tosca cookies.

MAKES APPROXIMATELY 18 COOKIES

14 cup melted butter

a quarter cup of honey or coconut syrup

14 cup oats (gluten-free)

a quarter cup of almond flour

coconut sugar (three tablespoons)

12 teaspoon vanilla extract

a quarter teaspoon of salt

2 tablespoons orange zest, grated (optional)

Preheat the oven to 400 degrees Fahrenheit. Use parchment paper or a silicone baking mat to line a baking pan.

In a saucepan, melt the butter and honey together until smooth. Remove the pan from the heat and stir in the oats, almond flour, coconut sugar, vanilla, salt, and, if desired, orange zest. Mix thoroughly. Dollop in teaspoon-sized dabs onto the prepared baking sheet. Allow lots of space around each cookie because they will spread a lot. Bake for about 8 minutes, or until golden brown. They'll burn easily, so keep an eye on them; undercooked cookies, on the other hand, will be too floppy. Allow them to cool and firm up before serving.

Chapter Two

COOKIES WITH NUTS AND BANANAS

These cookies are enjoyable to create and eat, especially for children. The combination of banana and nut is tempting.

MAKES APPROXIMATELY 10 COOKIES

113 cup mixed nuts (cashews, pecans, and/or walnuts)

2 peeled and sliced ripe bananas

1 teaspoon vanilla extract

12 teaspoon cinnamon powder

14 teaspoon cardamom powder

a quarter teaspoon of salt

a pinch of raisins

Preheat the oven to 350 degrees Fahrenheit and prepare a baking sheet with parchment paper. To make a coarse crumble, mix the nuts in a blender. Toss in the bananas. Continue blending in the vanilla, cinnamon, cardamom, and salt. Add the raisins and mix well. Roll tablespoonfuls of dough into balls and pat into 14-inch-thick cookies. Place on the baking sheet that has been prepared. Preheat oven to 350°F and bake for 20 minutes. After around 15 minutes, rotate the cookies to avoid scorching. Allow to cool before serving.

Chapter Three

HAZELNUT COOKIES WITH CACAO FILLING

With time, these chocolate-filled pastries improve. Tip: If you double the amount of filling and use it to frost each cookie individually, you may quadruple the number of cookies.

YIELDS 6–8 COOKIES

COOKIES

1 cup ground hazelnuts or hazelnut flour

14 cup oat flour or gluten-free oats, ground

12 cup cacao powder (raw)

1 teaspoon powdered baking soda

1 teaspoon powdered vanilla

1 egg, beaten or 2 tablespoons tapioca starch

a quarter teaspoon of salt

12 cup of butter (or coconut oil)

5–7 tbsp. honey or coconut nectar

FILLING

a quarter cup of nut butter

a third of a cup of coconut oil

2 tblsp cacao powder (raw)

3 tbsp. honey or coconut nectar

12 teaspoon extract de vanille

COOKIES. Preheat the oven to 350 degrees Fahrenheit and place a rack in the middle. Using parchment paper, line a baking sheet. Combine the nut flour, oat flour, cacao powder, baking powder, vanilla powder, tapioca starch (if using), and salt in a mixing dish. In the top of a double boiler, melt the butter until it's a runny consistency, then stir in the honey. If using, add the egg. Combine the wet and dry ingredients in a mixing bowl. Scoop the dough into tablespoonfuls, roll into balls, and flatten into 38-inch-thick cookies. Preheat oven to 350°F and bake for 10 minutes. (Be careful not to overbake the cookies, or they will become dry.) Prepare the filling while the cookies are baking.

FILLING. In the top of a double boiler, melt the nut butter and coconut oil. Mix in the cacao powder, honey, and vanilla extract until thoroughly combined. Put the spread in the fridge for a few minutes if it's too runny.

Remove the cookies from the oven and set aside to cool fully. Spread some filling between pairs of cookies to make double-decker cookies. Serve and have fun. Keep refrigerated.

Chapter Four

CHOCOLATE MUFFINS WITH CRUNCHY

The raw cacao nibs give these rich chocolate muffins a delightful crunch. I get a lot of compliments on these from other people, as well as from myself.

YIELDS 8–10 MUFFINS

MUFFINS

a total of 112 cup almond flour

12 cup cacao powder (raw)

13 cup honey or 14 cup coconut sugar

2 tablespoons powdered baking soda

3 beaten eggs

12 cup melted butter and/or coconut oil

12 cup oat milk, other milk substitute (see recipe), or coconut water + additional if necessary

vanilla extract (two teaspoons)

a pinch of salt

14 cup cacao nibs (raw)

Chocolate Icing Made Simple (see recipe or 129)

ABOVE ALL

Coconut flakes or desiccated coconut

MUFFINS. Preheat the oven to 350 degrees Fahrenheit and fill muffin tins with paper liners. In a single bowl, combine the almond flour, cacao powder, coconut sugar, and baking powder. Combine the eggs, butter, oat milk, vanilla essence, and salt in a separate bowl. Combine the wet and dry ingredients in a large mixing bowl. Add the raw cacao nibs and mix well. The dough should now be soft and spoonable, but not too liquid. If it's too dry, add a splash of oat milk. Fill muffin tins halfway with dough and bake for 25–35 minutes in the centre of the oven. The muffins should be somewhat soft in the middle. Allow the muffins to cool completely before frosting.

Prepare and spread the frosting on the muffins. Coconut should be sprinkled on top. Serve and have fun!

!

MOCHA MUFFINS WITH NUT BUTTER

Maiju, a friend of mine, is a huge foodie, especially when it comes to sweets. I frequently put my recipes to the test on her. When she hid a package of muffins from the other visitors after sampling them at a gathering, I knew they had passed with flying colours.

MAKES APPROXIMATELY 10 MUFFINS

MUFFINS

12 CUP CULTURED COCONUT FLOUR

14 cup cacao powder (raw)

2 tablespoons powdered baking soda

a third of a cup of honey or coconut syrup

4 big beaten eggs

12 cup heated coconut oil

12 cup oat milk or other milk substitute (recipe below) + extra if necessary

1 teaspoon extract de vanille

a third of a cup of strong coffee

ICING

12 cup coconut oil or butter

12 cup peanut butter (unsweetened)

a quarter-cup of coconut syrup

1 teaspoon extract de vanille

2 tbsp. oat milk (or other milk substitute) (see recipe)

MUFFINS. Preheat the oven to 400 degrees Fahrenheit. In a single dish, combine the coconut flour, cacao powder, and baking powder. Combine the honey, eggs, coconut oil, oat milk, and vanilla extract in a separate bowl. Pour the liquid into the dry ingredients and stir thoroughly. Mix in the coffee and set aside for about 5 minutes. The dough should have a soft, spoonable texture. If it's too dry, add a splash of oat milk. Fill muffin tins halfway with batter and bake for 20 minutes in the centre of the oven. The muffins should be somewhat soft in the middle. Allow the muffins to cool completely before frosting.

ICING. In a medium saucepan, melt the butter, peanut butter, and honey until smooth. Combine the vanilla essence and oat milk in a mixing bowl. Remove the pan from the heat and set aside a couple of teaspoons of the mixture. Place the leftover mixture in a basin and chill for a few minutes. To make a fluffy and light frosting, use a blender. Spread a large amount over the cooled muffins. Thin the reserved icing with a little oat milk, spoon it into a piping bag, and use it to finish decorating. Serve and have fun!

Chapter Five

DONUTS WITH CARAMEL

When I was a teenager, my favourite treat was caramel doughnuts, but my mother would only allow me to have them on rare occasions. Now I have an excellent substitute that I can eat without feeling guilty about!

MAKES APPROXIMATELY 8 DONUTS

DONUTS

14 cup melted butter or coconut oil + extra for greasing

a total of 112 cup almond flour

1 teaspoon powdered baking soda

a third of a cup of honey or coconut syrup

a quarter teaspoon of almond extract

12 teaspoon extract de vanille

apple cider vinegar, 1 teaspoon

4 egg whites, big

ICING WITH CARAMEL

Spreadable Caramel (see recipe)

2 tblsp almond butter (or other nut butter)

ABOVE ALL

walnuts, crushed

DONUTS. Preheat the oven to 350 degrees Fahrenheit and place a rack in the middle. Preheat the oven to 350°F and grease a doughnut pan. In a mixing bowl, combine the almond flour and baking powder. Combine the butter, honey, almond and vanilla extracts, and vinegar in a separate bowl. Mix the wet and dry ingredients together thoroughly.

Egg whites should be beaten until frothy in a clean basin. Carefully fold in the remaining ingredients. Evenly distribute the batter among the doughnut shapes. Bake for 15 minutes, or until golden brown. Remove the donuts from the pan once they have cooled.

ICING. Combine the caramel spread and almond butter in a mixing bowl. This icing should be poured over the donuts. Enjoy with a sprinkling of crumbled walnuts.

CINNAMON CHOCOLATE DONUTS A chocolate donut always works, no matter what the situation, where you are, or who you are. These delightful chocolate rounds are no exception.

MAKES APPROXIMATELY 8 DONUTS

DONUTS

14 cup coconut oil + more for frying

a quarter cup of coconut flour

12 CUP ALMONDFILLER

13 cup cacao powder (raw)

1 teaspoon powdered baking soda

1 teaspoon cinnamon powder

a quarter teaspoon of salt

three eggs

a third of a cup of honey or coconut syrup

apple cider vinegar, 1 teaspoon

1 teaspoon extract de vanille

Chocolate Icing Made Simple (see recipe or 129)

ABOVE ALL

walnuts, crushed

flakes of coconut

Preheat the oven to 350 degrees Fahrenheit and place a rack in the middle. Preheat the oven to 350°F and grease a doughnut pan. In a mixing dish, combine the flours, cacao powder, baking powder, cinnamon, and salt. Using two clean bowls, separate the egg yolks and whites. Add the honey, apple cider vinegar, vanilla extract, and 14 cup coconut oil to the bowl with the yolks. Join your hands and beat together. Combine the wet and dry ingredients in a mixing bowl. Whisk the egg whites until frothy, then fold them in with the rest of the ingredients. Distribute evenly amongst the donut moulds. Bake for 10–15 minutes, or until golden. Remove the donuts from the pan once they have cooled.

Make the icing and drizzle it over the doughnuts. Serve with a topping of crushed walnuts and coconut flakes.

Chapter Six

DONUTS WITH CARDAMOM AND VANILLA

Vegan vanilla donuts are a lovely and delicate snack. It's ideal for a Sunday treat or just before a sleep.

MAKES APPROXIMATELY 8 DONUTS

Greasing using coconut oil

3 tablespoons ground flaxseed + 13 cup warm water = 1 giant "flaxseed egg"

1 pound of rice flour

a third of a cup of potato flour

2 tablespoons powdered baking soda

psyllium husk powder or xanthan gum (12 teaspoon)

12 teaspoon cardamom powder

1 peeled ripe banana

1 gallon rice milk

3 tablespoons melted butter or coconut oil

14 cup honey + 1 teaspoon vanilla extract, or 12 teaspoon vanilla stevia

VANILLA WHITE CHOCOLATE ICING

12 cup cacao butter, grated

coconut oil (three tablespoons)

12 tsp vanilla stevia, honey, or vanilla essence

3 tbsp rice milk (or other milk substitute) (see recipe)

ABOVE ALL

Rice flour and/or puffed rice

Preheat the oven to 350 degrees Fahrenheit and place a rack in the middle. Preheat the oven to 350°F and grease a doughnut pan. Mix the flaxseeds with the water and set aside for 5–10 minutes to make the "flaxseed egg."

Combine the flours, baking powder, psyllium husk powder, and cardamom in a mixing bowl. In a separate bowl, mash the banana and stir in the rice milk, "flaxseed egg," and melted butter. Use the vanilla stevia to sweeten. Mix in the dry ingredients from the other bowl until a batter forms. Spoon the batter into the doughnut pan, dividing it equally, and bake for 25 minutes, or until slightly golden. Allow to cool after removing from the oven. Assemble the frosting.

ICING. In the top of a double boiler, melt the cacao butter and coconut oil. Combine the sweetener and rice milk in a mixing bowl. Transfer the bowl to an ice bath and whisk the mixture with a spoon until it thickens. You can also chill the mixture to set it, but don't leave it there for too long or it will become too rigid. Pour the frosting over the donuts that have been allowed to cool, then sprinkle with puffed rice or dust with rice flour using a sieve. Serve and have fun.

Chapter Seven

MARZIPAN BUNS WITH ORANGE FLOWERS

All sticky-bun devotees should try these marzipan-filled dream rolls. In place of the orange marzipan, you can fill these with the Caramel Spread from the recipe.

MAKES APPROXIMATELY 12 BUNS

BUNS

12 cup melted butter or coconut oil

12 CUP COCONUT SUCTION

2 eggs, big

14 cup almond milk (or another milk substitute) (see recipe)

1 cup flour made from almonds

1 cup flour made from buckwheat

psyllium husk powder, 112 teaspoons

1 teaspoon powdered baking soda

1 tblsp. cardamom powder

1 teaspoon cinnamon powder

a quarter teaspoon of salt

FILLING FOR ORANGE MARZIPAN

Make a double batch of Orange Marzipan (recipe below), with liquids doubled.

2 tblsp. orange blossom water

ABOVE ALL

Brushing with an egg that has been beaten (optional)

Sugar made from coconut

almonds, flakes

BUNS. Preheat the oven to 425 degrees Fahrenheit and place a rack in the middle. Using paper muffin liners, line a muffin tray. In a mixing bowl, combine the butter, coconut sugar, eggs, and almond milk. Combine the flours, psyllium husk powder, and baking powder in a separate bowl. Combine the cardamom, cinnamon, and salt in a bowl. Bit by little, stir the dry ingredients into the wet components. Allow the dough to rise for 10 minutes. Like other bun doughs, the dough should be easily moldable. Concentrate on preparing the filler.

FILLING. Make the orange marzipan as directed in the recipe, double the recipe, doubling the liquids again, and adding the orange flower water. (The extra liquids make it easier to distribute the marzipan.)

Roll the dough between two sheets of parchment paper into a rectangular shape with a rolling pin. Put the dough in the freezer for a few minutes if it's too difficult to deal with. This will make it easier to deal with. Fill the dough with a generous amount of marzipan filling. Roll the parchment paper into a large roll with the help of the parchment paper. Cut crosswise into 1 inch thick buns with a sharp knife. Place the buns in the prepared muffin pans, brush with beaten egg if desired, and top with flaked almonds and a pinch of coconut sugar. Bake for 10–15 minutes, or until slightly browned. Avoid baking the buns for too long if you want them to stay moist. The centres should be a little gooey. Remove from the oven, set aside to cool for a few minutes before serving.

Chapter Eight

SORBETS & ICE CREAMS

ICE CREAM WITH LICORICE

In the summer, I couldn't get the thought of licorice ice cream out of my head. I finally got the treat I sought after a few tries. When we tested this ice cream, the entire party fell in love with it. It's worthwhile to pursue your aspirations!

MAKES APPROXIMATELY 1 PINT

BASE OF ICE CREAM

2 organic eggs, big

a third of a cup of honey or coconut syrup

Coconut Whipped Cream (see recipe)

SAUCE WITH LICORICE

13 cup honey or dark coconut syrup

licorice powder, 2 tblsp.

BASE OF ICE CREAM In a mixing basin, whisk together the eggs and honey until frothy. With a rubber spatula, incorporate the whipped coconut cream into the egg mixture.

SAUCE WITH LICORICE. To make a smooth paste, combine the coconut syrup and licorice powder.

Fill an ice cream maker halfway with the ice cream base and follow the manufacturer's directions. Pour in the licorice sauce right before serving to form stripes in the ice cream. (If you don't have an ice cream machine, pour the mixture into a rimmed baking dish and place it in the freezer for 3 hours.) Stir every 45 minutes or so, and add the licorice sauce halfway through the freezing process.)

Chapter Nine

ICE CREAM WITH CARDAMOM AND PEACHES

Fresh peaches baked in the oven produce a delicious ice cream. It's even better if you serve it in a homemade waffle cone.

MAKES APPROXIMATELY 1 PINT

BASE OF ICE CREAM

3 peeled and pitted fresh peaches

13 cup honey or other sweetener of choice (maple syrup, for example)

1 teaspoon cardamom powder

1 teaspoon cinnamon powder

2 egg whites, big

2 full-fat coconut milk cans (13.5 oz each), refrigerated overnight

CONES OF WAFFLE (MAKES ABOUT 5)

2 egg whites, organic

14 cup melted and cooled butter or coconut oil + extra for greasing

12 c. coconut sugar + 12 c. vanilla stevia

12 cup rice flour (about)

1 teaspoon powdered psyllium husk

12 teaspoon vanilla extract

a pinch of salt

5 tbsp. oat milk (or other milk substitute) (see recipe)

Greasing using coconut oil

For the waffle moulds, use aluminium foil or cardboard.

BASE OF ICE CREAM Preheat the oven to 400 degrees Fahrenheit. Toss the peaches with the honey, cardamom, and cinnamon in a mixing bowl. Mix thoroughly. Bake for 20 minutes after pouring the mixture into a baking dish. Allow to cool.

Using an electric mixer, whip the egg whites until they are frothy. In a separate dish, make whipped coconut cream using the cans of coconut milk as directed on the recipe, eliminating the added sugars. Purée the roasted peaches in a blender. Depending on your desire, you can blend them smooth or leave them in lumps. Some of the purée should be saved for drizzling over the ice cream. Combine the peach purée, whipped coconut cream, and egg white foam in a mixing bowl. Fill an ice cream maker halfway with this ice cream foundation and follow the manufacturer's directions. (If you don't have an ice cream maker, pour the mixture into a rimmed baking dish and place in the freezer for about 2 hours.) Using a hand blender or handheld mixer, aggressively beat the mixture every 45 minutes.)

CONES OF WAFFLE In a clean basin, place the egg whites. Beat in the butter until it foams up. Combine the coconut sugar, rice flour, psyllium husk powder, vanilla powder, and salt in a mixing bowl and whisk slowly while adding to the butter mixture. Allow for 5 minutes after adding the oat milk. Cone shapes can be made out of foil or cardboard. A waffle iron should be preheated and greased. Fill the iron with a thin layer of the mixture, seal it, and bake for 2–3 minutes. The crispier the waffle cones are, the thinner the layer and the longer you bake them. Using a spatula, remove the waffle and roll it over the cone mould. Allow to cool before removing from the mould and drying on a wire rack. Rep with the rest of the batter.

Scoop the ice cream into balls and serve in the cones with the peach purée that was set aside.

Chapter Ten

CAKE WITH MANGO AND MELON SORBET

My family's favourite summer treat is this sorbet cake. Blend the frozen fruits till smooth, then add the toasted nuts and scoop into balls to speed up the process. It's great in both directions!

MAKES APPROXIMATELY 4 SERVINGS

2 peeled and pitted ripe mangos

12 cantaloupe or honeydew melon, peeled and seeded

1 peeled ripe banana

BASE FOR THE CAKE

macadamia nuts (12 cup)

12 c. almonds

4 pitted and sliced fresh dates

Greasing using coconut oil

2 tbsp. honey or coconut nectar

1 tbsp extract de vanille

ALMONDS ROASTED IN HONEY

a quarter cup of almonds

honey (two tablespoons)

coconut oil (two tablespoons)

SIZE OF TART PAN

8 and a half inches

Mango, melon, and banana should be diced and frozen overnight in an airtight container.

BASE FOR THE CAKE In a high-powered blender or food processor, grind the nuts. Blend in the dates until you have a moldable dough. Grease a removable-base high-sided tart pan and press the dough into it.

Blend the frozen fruits in a blender until they form a sorbet-like consistency. (Save a couple of spoonfuls of sliced mango for later.) Blend in the honey and vanilla extract. Place the pan in the freezer for 3 hours to solidify the sorbet mixture on top of the cake base.

ALMONDS ROASTED IN HONEY. In a mortar and pestle, crush some of the almonds. In a saucepan, combine the honey and coconut oil, then add the crushed and whole almonds, tossing and cooking lightly until they begin to brown. Invert the sorbet cake onto a plate, then onto a serving platter again. Place the roasted almonds on top. Serve and savour right now!

ICE CREAM WITH COOKIES AND SALTED PEANUTS

These are for you if you like sweet and salty flavours, as well as nut butter. You won't forget the delicious combination of soft-textured cookies and chocolate ice cream rolled in salted peanuts. Keep the leftover cookies in the freezer for later use.

MAKES APPROXIMATELY 6 SERVINGS

CREAM OF ICE

1 pound cashews

1 banana, ripe

1 dropperful chocolate stevia or 13 cup honey

coconut oil (three tablespoons)

12 cup coconut milk (full-fat) + additional as needed

14 cup cacao powder (raw)

CUPCAKES (MAKES ABOUT 16)

1 cup flour made from almonds

a third of a cup of coconut flour

1 tablespoon powdered psyllium husk

1 teaspoon powdered baking soda

a pinch of salt

a third of a cup of honey or coconut syrup

13 cup nut butter (peanut or otherwise)

a third of a cup of coconut oil

2 eggs, big

12 teaspoon extract de vanille

1 cup oat milk (or another milk substitute) (see recipe)

ABOVE ALL

peanuts, salted, ground

CREAM OF ICE. Combine the cashews, banana, honey, coconut oil, coconut milk, and cacao powder in a high-powered blender or food processor. To make a smooth, thick concoction, combine all of the ingredients in a blender. If the mixture isn't smooth enough, add a splash of coconut milk. Taste and adjust the seasonings as needed. Fill the ice cream maker halfway with the mixture and process according to the manufacturer's instructions. (Alternatively, pour into a rimmed baking dish and place in the freezer for 3–4 hours.) To keep the ice cream frothy, stir every 45 minutes to break up the ice crystals.) Meanwhile, the cookies must be prepared.

COOKIES. Preheat the oven to 350 degrees Fahrenheit and prepare a baking sheet with parchment paper. In a mixing dish, combine the flours, psyllium husk powder, baking powder, and salt. In the top of a double boiler, melt the honey, peanut butter, and coconut oil. Add the eggs and vanilla essence to this mixture in a separate bowl. To make a fluffy mixture, combine all of the ingredients in a mixing bowl. Continue mixing while adding the dry ingredients. Mix in the oat milk until a dough forms.

Take a tablespoon of dough at a time, roll it into a ball, and set it on the baking sheet that has been prepared. Press the balls into flat biscuits with damp palms. Preheat oven to 350°F and bake for 12 minutes. Allow the cookies to cool completely on a wire rack.

ASSEMBLY. Make little balls of ice cream and sandwich them between two cookies. Roll the ice cream cookies with salted peanuts on all sides. Serve immediately or store in the freezer until ready to use.

Chapter Eleven

DREAMSICLES WITH ARTISANAL INGREDIENTS

In Popsicle moulds, make these delectable homemade chocolate ice pops. You may make the icing from scratch or just use a melted raw chocolate bar with some crushed nuts.

MAKES APPROXIMATELY 4 SERVINGS

CREAM OF ICE

2 peeled and sliced ripe bananas

nut butter (about 2 tablespoons)

a quarter cup of almonds

5 tbsp. liquid

2 tblsp cacao nibs (raw)

1 tbsp. honey or coconut nectar

12 tsp vanilla extract

CHOCOLATE CREAM CREAM CREAM CREAM CREAM CR

13 cup cacao butter, grated

coconut oil (two tablespoons)

14 cup cacao powder (raw)

1 tbsp. honey or coconut nectar

a little teaspoon of salt

ABOVE ALL

nuts that have been crushed (optional)

CREAM OF ICE. Blend the bananas, nut butter, and almonds in a high-powered blender or food processor until smooth and thick, adding just enough water to achieve the desired consistency. (If you use too much water, the ice cream will crystallise.) Combine the cacao nibs, honey, and vanilla powder in a mixing bowl. Pulse to combine, breaking up the cacao nibs as you go. Fill ice pop moulds halfway with the mixture and freeze for a few hours. Prepare the icing right before you're ready to serve.

ICING. In the top of a double boiler, melt the cacao butter and coconut oil. Combine the cacao powder, honey, and salt in a mixing bowl. Remove the ice pops from the freezer and coat them in chocolate frosting with a spoon. If desired, sprinkle the crumbled nuts on top. Serve right away, or keep on a dish in the freezer.

Chapter Twelve

ICE CREAM WITH CHERRY AND CHOCOLATE

Though you can only taste the cherries and chocolate in this sinfully delicious cherry-studded chocolate ice cream, hemp seeds are a surprising healthy component.

MAKES APPROXIMATELY 1 PINT

13 cup chopped cherries + 1 cup pitted whole fresh cherries

2 teaspoons melted coconut oil

a third of a cup of honey or coconut sugar

1 teaspoon extract de vanille

12 CUP HORSEWEED SEEDS

13 cup cacao powder (raw)

As needed, use water or a milk substitute (see recipe).

14 cup (2 ounces) bought or handmade ground raw chocolate (see Basic Chocolate, see recipe)

In a high-powered blender or food processor, combine the 1 cup cherries, coconut oil, honey, and vanilla essence. Add the hemp seeds, cacao powder, and a splash of water if necessary to achieve a smooth consistency. Stir in the 13 cup chopped cherries and the raw chocolate using a spoon.

Pour the mixture into an ice cream machine and follow the manufacturer's directions for making ice cream. (If you don't have an ice cream maker, pour the mixture onto a rimmed baking dish and place it in the freezer for a few hours.) To keep the ice cream frothy, mix thoroughly every 45 minutes.)

Scoop the ice cream into balls when it's done, serve, and enjoy!

Chapter Thirteen

SQUARES ESKIMO

Vanilla ice cream is one of life's simple pleasures. This ice cream recipe is a tribute to two of life's most essential ingredients: vanilla ice cream and chocolate.

MAKES APPROXIMATELY 6 SERVINGS

CREAM OF ICE

12 cup cashews, soaked for one hour

macadamia nuts (12 cup)

12 cup oat milk (or other milk substitute) (see recipe)

13 cup melted coconut oil

honey (two tablespoons)

1 tbsp extract de vanille

8 stevia drops, or as needed

Easy Chocolate Icing in a Double Batch (see recipe or 129)

SIZE OF THE CONTAINER

Approximately 5 x 10 inches

CREAM OF ICE. Drain and rinse the soaked nuts before combining them with the oat milk in a high-powered blender or food processor. To make a smooth concoction, combine all of the ingredients in a blender. Combine the coconut oil, honey, vanilla essence, and stevia in a mixing bowl. Blend until completely smooth. Pour the mixture into a high-sided dish lined with plastic wrap or parchment paper, allowing it to dangle over the sides. Freeze for 3 hours or until solid. Remove the ice cream from the container and cut it into squares. Place the squares back in the freezer.

Make two batches of a simple chocolate icing.

Remove the squares from the freezer and dip each one into the chocolate icing one at a time. You can also use a spoon to coat the squares in chocolate. Place on a parchment paper-lined serving platter and freeze until ready to serve.

TIP! If you want to maintain the ice cream filling's colour white, use light honey and stevia as sweeteners.

Chapter Fourteen

ICE CREAM WITH STRAWBERRY AND ROSE

Strawberry and rose are a match made in heaven. They complement each other well in ice cream.

MAKES APPROXIMATELY 1 PINT

CREAM OF ICE

12 cup strawberries, fresh or frozen

1 peeled and sliced ripe banana

1 cup coconut milk (full fat)

12 teaspoon vanilla extract

1 teaspoon rose essential oil

3 egg whites, big

CHOCOLATE CREAM CREAM CREAM CREAM CREAM CR

12 cup Basic Chocolate or 4 ounces unsweetened dark or raw chocolate, purchased or homemade (see recipe)

Set aside about a quarter cup of strawberries. Pour the remaining ingredients into a blender. Blend together the banana, coconut milk, vanilla powder, and rose extract until creamy.

In a mixing bowl, whisk the egg whites until stiff and glossy peaks form. Combine the strawberry mixture and fold it in. With kitchen scissors, cut the remaining strawberries into the bowl and fold them in. If desired, taste and adjust the sweetness. Make ice cream with the mixture according to the directions on your ice cream maker. Alternatively, you can freeze the bowl for 30–45 minutes, stirring every 30–45 minutes.

Make a frosting or eat it plain. Melt the raw or unsweetened dark chocolate in the top of a double boiler, or use the Basic Chocolate. Make ice cream balls and dip them in melted chocolate. The chocolate will quickly set over the cold ice cream. Serve and have fun!

Replace the egg whites with 13 cup macadamia nuts and 2 tbsp heated coconut oil for a vegan alternative.

Chapter Fifteen

ICE CREAM CAKE TIRAMISU

Originally, I planned to include this recipe with the cakes because this cake keeps well in the refrigerator. It is, however, finest when frozen and then gently thawed.

YIELDS SIX SERVINGS

FILLING WITH CREAM

macadamia nuts, 2 cups

112 cup almond milk (or other milk substitute) (see recipe)

a third of a cup of honey or coconut syrup

1 tbsp extract de vanille

12 cup cacao butter, grated

a third of a cup of coconut oil

LAYER OF CAKE

1 pound of oat flakes

12 cup raisins (soft)

2 pitted fresh dates

3 teaspoons melted coconut oil

a quarter-cup of strong coffee

14 cup liqueur d'amandes

1 tablespoon cacao powder (raw)

honey (three tablespoons)

1 teaspoon extract de vanille

1 teaspoon of salt

ABOVE ALL

Coconut Whipped Cream (see recipe)

Cacao powder (raw)

SIZE OF THE CONTAINER

Approximately 5 x 8 inches

FILLING WITH CREAM. Blend the nuts and almond milk until smooth in a high-powered blender or food processor. Combine the honey and vanilla extract in a mixing bowl. In the top of a double boiler, melt the cacao butter and coconut oil. Combine this mixture with the remaining ingredients in a blender and blend until smooth. If desired, taste and adjust the sweetness or flavourings. Half of the mixture should be poured into a high-sided rectangle dish and frozen for 30 minutes. Reserve the remainder in a basin. Prepare the top layer of the cake.

LAYER OF CAKE. Blend the oat flakes, raisins, dates, coconut oil, coffee, and liqueur together into a dough in a blender. Combine the cacao powder, honey, vanilla extract, and salt in a mixing bowl. Mix thoroughly. Taste and adjust the seasonings as needed.

Bring the dish out of the freezer once the cream filling has solidified a little and spoon half of the cake layer on top. Over the cake layer, pour the reserved cream filling. Return the surface to the freezer until it has hardened. Return to the freezer for a few hours after removing the last cake layer and spooning it on top.

Whip the coconut cream until it is light and fluffy. Remove the dish from the freezer and invert it onto a baking sheet to unmold the cake. Decorate the cake with whipped coconut cream in a piping bag. Cacao powder is sprinkled on top. Serve immediately or store in the freezer until ready to use.

Chapter Sixteen

BUTTER WITH VANILLA COCONUT

SPREADS, JAMS, AND GARNISHES

This coconut butter can be used in baking, as a spread, or as a dessert frosting. Because it's a little sweet, you might want to reduce the other sweeteners.

MAKES APPROXIMATELY 1 CUP

2 cups flakes de coco

1 teaspoon vanilla extract

In a high-powered blender or food processor, crush the coconut flakes to a flour-like consistency on medium speed. Continue to run the machine until the mixture becomes sticky and gritty. Scrape the mixture from the sides of the bowl to the middle using a rubber spatula if necessary. Turn the machine on full speed when the mixture begins to resemble butter to make the mixture as smooth as possible. Depending on the power of your machine, making coconut butter might take anywhere from 1 to 5 minutes. Mix in the vanilla powder lightly. To keep the coconut butter, use a glass jar with a tight-fitting cover. At room temperature, it will keep for several weeks. Keep it out of the fridge since it will be difficult to distribute. (To soften hardened coconut butter, use a double boiler.)

Chapter Seventeen

BUTTER OF ALMOND CHOCOLATE

Nut and almond butters can be used as a spread, in baked goods, as frosting, and in a variety of other ways. Different nuts can be substituted for the almonds, and the chocolate can be omitted.

MAKES APPROXIMATELY 1 CUP

Almonds, blanched, 112 cup

1 tbsp almond butter (optional)

3 tblsp cacao powder (raw)

1 tablespoon melted coconut oil

3 tbsp. honey or coconut nectar

a pinch of salt

In a high-powered blender or food processor, combine the almonds. Grind into a fine flour and continue to combine until the almond powder begins to resemble wax. If necessary, add a few drops of almond oil; however, if you have a powerful blender, you can prepare almond butter without it. Blend till the mixture turns into almond butter. It will take roughly 15 minutes to complete the operation. Combine the cacao powder, coconut oil, honey, and salt in a mixing bowl. Mix thoroughly.

2 CHOCOLATE ICING EASY

Choose from two simple chocolate icings to use as fillings or icings for baked products.

CHOCOLATE DATE ICING

MAKES APPROXIMATELY 12 CUP

12 cup pitted fresh dates

13 cup melted coconut oil

13 cup cacao powder (raw)

a third of a cup of water, or as needed

Blend the dates and melted coconut oil until smooth in a blender. Add the cacao powder and continue to run the machine, adding water in small increments until you reach the desired thickness. Serve as a filling or frosting.

The sole stipulation for success is that the dates are soft and juicy. The best dates are Medjool dates. Soak the dates for about an hour if they feel dry.

CHOCOLATE AVOCADO ICING

MAKES APPROXIMATELY 1 CUP

1 tbsp raw cacao butter, ground

coconut oil (two tablespoons)

13 cup of honey

13 cup cacao powder (raw)

2 pitted and halved ripe avocados

Melt the cacao butter, coconut oil, and honey in the top of a double boiler. Add the cacao powder to the mix. In a blender, chop and scoop the avocados, then add the melted cacao mixture. Blend until completely smooth.

SPREAD WITH CARAMEL

As an icing, a filling, an ice cream topping, a dip, or a spread, use this caramel sauce. The best dates for this recipe are soft Medjool dates.

MAKES APPROXIMATELY 1 CUP

15–20 brand-new dates

coconut oil (two tablespoons)

12 teaspoon extract de vanille

a quarter teaspoon of salt

1–5 tbsp. of water

Dates should be pitted. Remove the peels as well if you want the caramel to be really soft and don’t know how powerful your blender is. (Under running water, peeling fresh dates is simple.) Blend the dates and coconut oil together in a blender until smooth. Mix in the vanilla extract and salt once more. Pour in just enough water to form a smooth, runny purée. Fill a glass jar halfway with caramel sauce and close tightly. Keep refrigerated.

Chapter Eighteen

COCONUT CREAM WITH WHIPPING

This is a fantastic substitute for classic whipped cream in baked goods and icings. It's worth noting that coconut milk manufacturers vary: some make thick whipped cream readily, while others don't. Try a few different brands until you discover one that you like.

MAKES APPROXIMATELY 2 CUPS

2 full-fat coconut milk cans (13.5 oz each), refrigerated overnight

honey or coconut syrup, 1–2 teaspoons

12 teaspoon vanilla extract

Drain the clear liquid from the bottom of the two coconut milk cans. (Save this liquid for something else, like a smoothie.) Fill a bowl halfway with the thick coconut cream from the cans. Using an electric mixer, beat the mixture until it thickens. Lift the mixer regularly while mixing to aerate the cream and make it frothy. Combine the honey and vanilla powder in a mixing bowl. If the whipped coconut cream becomes too runny, place it in the refrigerator. As with regular whipped cream, use as icing or for decorating.

Give the can of coconut milk a good shake before using it. Don't buy that can if you hear splashing. Drop it in your basket if you hear a heavy slush.

Chapter Nineteen

BUTTER WITH PEANUTS

Use this spread as a filler or a topping for baked dishes and cakes. Vegans can substitute coconut oil for the butter and coconut syrup for the honey. In the fridge, the mixture will become pretty solid.

MAKES APPROXIMATELY 1 CUP

12 cup coconut oil or butter

12 cup peanut butter (unsweetened)

4 tbsp. honey or coconut nectar

1 tbsp extract de vanille

oat milk (3 tblsp) (see recipe)

Melt the butter, peanut butter, and honey together in a skillet over medium heat until smooth. Combine the vanilla essence and oat milk in a mixing bowl. Mix thoroughly. Remove the pan from the heat and transfer the contents to a mixing bowl. Refrigerate for approximately 15 minutes. Remove the bowl from the fridge and use an electric mixer to make a frothy, light spread.

Chapter Twenty

ALTERNATIVES TO MILK WITHOUT THE DAIRY

Who needs cow's milk when plant-based alternatives are so simple and inexpensive to make? You'll find your favourite by experimenting with different ingredients. Alternatives to milk are delicious to cook with and drink!

MILK OF ALMOND

MAKES APPROXIMATELY 2 CUPS

1 pound of almonds (soaked overnight in water to cover, if you like)

2 c. liquid

2 pitted and coarsely chopped fresh dates

12 teaspoon vanilla extract

In a blender, combine the almonds (soaked or not), water, and dates until smooth. To make the milk smooth, strain off the fibres with a colander coated with cheesecloth. Vanilla powder is added as a finishing touch. Keep refrigerated in an airtight bottle or jar. Within 4–5 days, drink. Before using, give it a good shake.

MILK FROM OATS

MAKES APPROXIMATELY 2 CUPS

1 pound of oat flakes

2 cups water (or more if necessary)

honey (two tablespoons)

12 teaspoon cinnamon powder

12 teaspoon vanilla extract

a quarter teaspoon of salt

Soak the oat flakes for 30 minutes after rinsing them. Rinse once more. In a blender, combine the 2 cups water. If you want your milk to be thinner, add additional water. For around 15 seconds, blend at high speed. Save the oat solids for subsequent baking by straining the milk. Rinse the blender and re-fill it with milk. Blend once more and strain. You can strain the milk however many times you like. Usually, three times is enough to smooth out the milk. During the last round of mixing, add the honey, cinnamon (if using), vanilla powder, and salt. Keep refrigerated in an airtight bottle or jar. Within 4–5 days, drink. Before usage, give it a good shake.

MILK FROM SESAME SEEDS

MAKES APPROXIMATELY 2 CUPS

1 cup sesame seeds, unhulled

4 pitted fresh dates

2 c. liquid

12 teaspoon vanilla extract

a quarter teaspoon of salt

Sesame seeds should be soaked for at least 6 hours or overnight. In a separate container, soak the dates. Sesame seeds should be drained and rinsed. In a blender, combine the water, drained sesame seeds, and dates. Blend for roughly 30 seconds at high speed. Strain. Add the vanilla and salt and stir. Keep refrigerated in an airtight bottle or jar. Within 4–5 days, drink. Before usage, give it a good shake.

Chapter Twenty-one

YOGURTS WITHOUT DAIRY

Coconut or almonds can be used to make delicate milk-free yoghurts.

YOGURT WITH COCONUT

MAKES APPROXIMATELY 1 CUP

1 can coconut milk, full fat, refrigerated overnight

2 pills of probiotics

honey (approximately 1–2 teaspoons)

12 teaspoon vanilla extract

Boiling water will sterilise a glass jar (or by washing it in a dishwasher). Carefully dry the glass. Scrape the white thick layer of coconut cream from the coconut milk can into the jar and top with as much coconut milk as needed to reach the desired consistency. 2 probiotic capsules, opened, powdered, poured into jar, and mixed with a spoon Toss in the honey. Cover the jar opening with a folded cheesecloth or other clean cloth and tighten it with a rubber band. Turn on the oven light but not the oven itself. Place the jar in the oven overnight to cool. The next day, add the vanilla extract and chill the yoghurt.

YOGURT WITH ALMONDS

MAKES APPROXIMATELY 112 CUPS

1 cup almonds, 1 hour soaking

1 cup oat milk (or another milk substitute) (see recipe)

2 pills of probiotics

honey (approximately 1–2 teaspoons)

12 teaspoon vanilla extract

Boiling water will sterilise a glass jar (or by washing it in a dishwasher). Carefully dry the glass. Place the soaked almonds in a blender after draining and rinsing them. Blend in the oat milk until it is completely smooth. Fill the container halfway with this mixture. 2 probiotic capsules, opened, powdered, poured into jar, and mixed with a spoon Add the honey and mix well. Cover the jar opening with a folded cheesecloth or other clean cloth and tighten it with a rubber band. Turn on the oven light but not the oven itself. Place the jar in the oven overnight to cool. The next day, add the vanilla extract and chill the yoghurt.

Warm the fluid slightly before adding the probiotic powder to speed up the fermentation process. Refrigerate the yoghurt and use it within a week. The yoghurt will thicken while it sits in the refrigerator.

Chapter Twenty-two

JAMS OF CHIA

Chia seeds naturally create a gel when they come into contact with water. Take advantage of this to make delicious jams. Experiment with different berries and fruits on their own or in combinations. Flaxseeds, which react similarly to water, can also be used to make jam.

RASPBERRY ROSE JAM

MAKES APPROXIMATELY 1 CUP

1 cup raspberries (fresh or frozen)

13 cup of honey

2 teaspoons rose extract or a small handful of organic rose petals

14 cup chia seeds or flaxseed powder, or as needed

In a blender, combine the raspberries, honey, and rose petals or extract. Purée until completely smooth, or leave some pieces in. Pour into an airtight glass container and stir in enough chia seeds to achieve the desired consistency. Refrigerate for at least one night. Use as a jam, a filling, or in any other way you'd like. Refrigerate for up to a week before using.

Because flaxseeds are a little firmer than chia seeds, I crush them first before putting them in jam.

Chapter Twenty-three

JAM WITH PEACHES AND LAVENDER

MAKES APPROXIMATELY 1 CUP

14 cup of water

2 tbsp lavender flowers (dry)

3 big pitted peaches

13 cup of honey

14 cup chia seeds or flaxseed powder

Bring the water to a boil and then pour over the lavender flowers. Allow for a 20-minute steep, then strain out the flowers and save the lavender water. Place the peaches in a blender and chop them up. Combine the lavender water and honey in a bowl. Blend. Fill a glass jar with the mixture and seal it. Add the chia seeds and mix well. Allow for at least 30 minutes of rest time, or overnight. Refrigerate for up to a week before using.

PUDDDING WITH ROASTED CASHEWS

YIELDS 6 SERVINGS

I have food cravings about as often as I breathe, and one of my favourites is cashews. I had a cashew fixation when I made this pudding; I would have eaten an old sock if it had cashews in it! This dish arose from my passion with cashews, which I learned are ideal for pudding. They're the richest, most delicious, and most delectable nut I've ever tasted, with a flavour that reminds me of a crock of butter with just a hint of delicate nuttiness. Don't wait for the cashews to cool before slicing them; putting them into the hot milk while they're still warm helps release their amazingly fragrant oils.

2 cups raw cashews, whole

1 14 gallon whole milk

a quarter-cup of heavy cream

12 cup of sugar

a third of a cup of cornstarch

3 beaten egg yolks

a quarter teaspoon of salt

1. Preheat the oven to 350 degrees Fahrenheit.

2. Roast cashews on a rimmed baking sheet for 7–8 minutes, or until gently brown and aromatic.

3. Place the heated cashews in a food processor and pulse 3–4 times until roughly chopped (do not overpulse or you'll end up with cashew paste), or place in a towel and crush with a rolling pin or wine bottle.

4. In a medium saucepan, simmer the milk, cream, and chopped cashews for 5–6 minutes, or until steaming but not boiling. Steep for at least 2 hours in the refrigerator; for optimum cashewness, steep overnight.

5. Pour the milk into a large measuring cup, straining off the cashews. To make a total of 212 cups liquid, add more milk if necessary.

6. In a medium saucepan, mix together the strained cashew milk and the additional ingredients vigorously.

7. Cook, whisking continually, for 5–6 minutes over medium-high heat, until mixture begins to thicken. (It's done when you can raise the whisk from the pudding and see a faint shadow.) The pudding will appear loose at first, but as it cools, it will thicken even more.)

8. Strain the pudding into a bowl through a fine-mesh sieve, pushing the pudding through with a spatula.

9. Allow it cool for 10 minutes at room temperature before pressing a layer of plastic wrap onto the surface and chilling for 2 hours.

PAIRINGS RECOMMENDED: Candied Mixed Nuts

Chapter Twenty-four

MY FAVOURITE RECIPES

YIELDS 6 SERVINGS

I'm a mint connoisseur who can trace my mint addiction all the way back to my home state of Ohio. Back in Cleveland, there's a fantastic ice cream shop called Pierre's, where the mint chocolate chip scoop is made up of thin chocolate shards rather than the annoying chocolate chips that freeze, harden, and chip your fillings. Arriving in New York and noticing the glaring lack of Pierre's gave me a new appreciation for a phrase I'd heard my whole life: "Desperate times call for desperate measures." So, once I discovered I was always sprinkling chocolate sprinkles on top of my usual mint pudding recipe, I gave in to the temptation of a Pierre's-style dessert.

1 14 gallon whole milk

a quarter-cup of heavy cream

1 fresh mint bunch, cleaned and dried

14 cup of sugar

a third of a cup of cornstarch

3 beaten egg yolks

a quarter teaspoon of salt

4 ounces chopped bittersweet chocolate (70 percent cocoa)

1. Heat milk and cream in a medium saucepan over medium heat until very hot but not boiling, about 4–5 minutes. Remove from heat, add mint, and steep for 20–30 minutes, or until cool to room temperature. Chill overnight or up to 24 hours in refrigerator.

2. Strain the milk and return it to the saucepan, removing the mint. Whisk together the sugar, cornstarch, egg yolks, and salt in a large mixing bowl.

3. Cook, whisking continually, for 5–6 minutes over medium-high heat, until mixture begins to thicken. (It's done when you can raise the whisk from the pudding and see a faint shadow.) The pudding will appear loose at first, but as it cools, it will thicken even more.)

4. Strain the pudding into a bowl through a fine-mesh sieve, squeezing the pudding through with a spatula.

5. Allow to cool for 10 minutes at room temperature before pressing a layer of plastic wrap onto the surface and chilling for 2 hours.

6. Preheat oven to 350°F and line a 9-by-9-inch square pan with parchment paper. Melt the chocolate in a double boiler until it is completely smooth. Pour onto prepared parchment-lined pan and freeze for 15–20 minutes, or until you have one paper-thin, solid piece of chocolate.

7. Break up the chocolate into shards with your hands and swirl them into the cold pudding until it resembles a Jackson Pollock painting.

PAIRING RECOMMENDED: Brownie Crumbs

6–8 SERVINGS

One of the desserts I had the honour of cooking while working in the kitchen at Daniel Boulud's DB Bistro Moderne was a tart fruit crémeux with hazelnut mousse and macarons. The dish was acidic but light, and I knew I had to recreate it in pudding form. This tangy and luscious passion fruit dessert is the outcome. Look for the purest, most concentrated juice you can find—the better the curd, the better the pudding!

CURD

12 cup pure passion fruit puree plus 2 teaspoons (available at specialty stores)

lemon juice (two teaspoons)

two eggs

2 beaten egg yolks

5 teaspoons melted butter

12 cup of sugar

a quarter teaspoon of salt

1 lemon, zested

PUDDING INSTRUCTIONS:

14 quarts milk

a quarter-cup of heavy cream

14 cup of sugar

a third of a cup of cornstarch

3 beaten egg yolks

a quarter teaspoon of salt

1 teaspoon extract de vanille

MAKE CURD CURD CURD CURD CURD CU

1. In a small saucepan, whisk together all of the ingredients over medium heat until the curd coats the back of a spoon, about 6–7 minutes. (Curd will appear to be a little loose.)

2. Strain the curd into a basin through a fine-mesh sieve, pushing the curd through with a silicone spatula.

3. Place a layer of plastic wrap on top of the curd and chill for 1 hour, or until fully cool.

HOW TO MAKE PUDDING:

1. In a medium saucepan, mix together all of the ingredients, except the vanilla extract, vigorously.

2. Cook, whisking continually, until the mixture is thick, 5–6 minutes over medium-high heat. (It's done when you can take the whisk from the pudding and see a shadow.)

3. Strain the pudding into a bowl through a fine-mesh sieve, squeezing the pudding through with a silicone spatula. Whisk in the vanilla extract.

4. Allow it cool for 10 minutes at room temperature before pressing a layer of plastic wrap onto the surface and chilling for 2 hours.

5. Once the curd and pudding are cold, whisk them together in a medium mixing bowl until fully combined.

6–8 SERVINGS PINEAPPLE CURD

I don't drink alcohol (trust me, I don't need it), but when everyone else is celebrating with a cocktail, I like to have a drink in my hand. A virgin pia colada is always my first choice—the creamy, fruity, tropical aromas never fail to entice me. I realised I was onto something when I started thinking about how to translate those flavours into a pudding. Here, pineapple curd is mixed into a super-creamy pudding, giving it a flavour that reminds me of a pineapple Creamsicle.

CURD CURD CURD CURD CURD CURD

3 cups pineapple juice (fresh or canned)

lemon juice (two teaspoons)

two eggs

2 beaten egg yolks

5 teaspoons melted butter

12 cup of sugar

a quarter teaspoon of salt

1 lemon, zested

PUDDING INSTRUCTIONS:

1 14 gallon whole milk

a quarter-cup of heavy cream

14 cup of sugar

a third of a cup of cornstarch

3 beaten egg yolks

a quarter teaspoon of salt

MAKE CURD CURD CURD CURD CURD CU

1. Bring the pineapple juice to a boil in a small saucepan over medium-high heat and cook for 20 minutes, or until the juice is reduced to 12 cup.

2. Stir in the other ingredients and simmer, stirring constantly, over medium heat for 6–7 minutes, or until the curd coats the back of a spoon.

3. Strain the curd into a bowl through a fine-mesh sieve, pushing the curd through the sieve with a spatula.

4. Press a layer of plastic wrap onto the surface of the curd and chill for 2 hours in the refrigerator.

HOW TO MAKE PUDDING:

1. In a medium saucepan, mix together all of the ingredients vigorously.

2. Cook, whisking continually, until the mixture is thick, 5–6 minutes over medium-high heat. (It's done when you can take the whisk from the pudding and see a shadow.)

3. Strain the pudding into a bowl through a fine-mesh sieve, squeezing the pudding through with a silicone spatula.

4. Allow it cool for 10 minutes at room temperature before pressing a layer of plastic wrap onto the surface and chilling for 2 hours.

5. Once the curd and pudding are cold, whisk them together in a medium mixing bowl until completely combined.

PAIRING SUGGESTIONS: Candied Mixed Nuts; Marshmallow Crème

Chapter Twenty-five

LIME JUICE PUDDING

YIELDS 6 SERVINGS

This pudding was made to accompany a Key lime pudding cheesecake, which is one of the shop's most popular desserts. Because of its pleasingly pucker-inducing sourness, even non-sweets individuals (do they exist?) enjoy this one. Key limes are small and sour, with a super-acidic yet slightly more flowery flavour than regular limes, often known as Persian limes. To extract the juice from the little green spheres, use a clamp-style citrus squeezer and fresh Key limes (they often come in a net bag because they're so small). If you can't locate them fresh, bottled Key lime juice is widely accessible. In a pinch, normal limes will suffice.

CURD

12 cup plus 2 tablespoons lime juice (key lime or normal)

two eggs

2 beaten egg yolks

5 teaspoons melted butter

12 cup of sugar

a quarter teaspoon of salt

3 key limes or 1 ordinary lime, zest

PUDDING INSTRUCTIONS:

1 14 gallon whole milk

a quarter-cup of heavy cream

14 cup of sugar

a third of a cup of cornstarch

a quarter teaspoon of salt

3 beaten egg yolks

1 teaspoon extract de vanille

MAKE CURD CURD CURD CURD CURD CU

1. Combine all ingredients in a small saucepan and whisk continually over medium heat for 4–5 minutes, or until curd coats the back of a spoon.

2. Strain the curd into a bowl through a fine-mesh sieve, pushing the curd through the sieve with a spatula.

3. Press a layer of plastic wrap across the curd's surface and chill for 1 hour in the refrigerator.

HOW TO MAKE PUDDING:

1. In a medium saucepan, whisk together all of the ingredients, except the vanilla extract, until smooth.

2. Cook, whisking continually, for 5–6 minutes over medium-high heat, until thickened. (It's done when you can take the whisk from the pudding and see a shadow.)

3. Strain the pudding into a bowl through a fine-mesh sieve, squeezing the pudding through with a spatula. Whisk in the vanilla extract.

4. Allow it cool for 10 minutes at room temperature before pressing a layer of plastic wrap onto the surface and chilling for 2 hours.

5. Once the curd and pudding are cold, whisk them together in a medium mixing bowl until completely combined.

GRAHAM CRUMBS AND WHIPPED CREAM ARE SUGGESTED PAIRINGS

Chapter Twenty-six

MAPLE PUDDING

4–6 SERVINGS

I spend the most of my waking hours at Puddin', where I work with a fantastic team that turns a job into a tight community. Someone will invariably have a bizarre food yearning, and it is in my nature to try to satisfy it. One of my employees expressed a desire for pancakes and syrup after thirteen hours of stirring pudding. The neurons in my pudding-obsessed brain started firing, and zing!—maple pudding was born. Use dark, intense grade B maple syrup for this recipe, as it has a remarkably complex flavour. You'll be able to discern all of the subtleties of the syrup if you stir it in near the end. Slowly drizzle in the syrup; if you do it too quickly, your pudding will become liquidy.

1 14 gallon whole milk

a quarter-cup of heavy cream

cornstarch (six tablespoons)

3 beaten egg yolks

14 cup sugar (dark brown)

a quarter teaspoon of salt

1 teaspoon extract de vanille

1 cup maple syrup (ideally grade B) of good quality

1. Whisk together the milk, cream, cornstarch, egg yolks, brown sugar, and salt vigorously in a medium saucepan.

2. Cook, whisking continually, for 5–6 minutes over medium heat, until the mixture is thick. (It's done when you can take the whisk from the pudding and it leaves a shadow; this pudding will appear thicker than others at first, but it will thin out once you add the maple syrup.)

3. Strain the pudding into a bowl through a fine-mesh sieve, squeezing the pudding through with a spatula. Whisk in the vanilla extract, then gradually drizzle in the maple syrup.

4. Allow it cool for 10 minutes at room temperature before pressing a layer of plastic wrap onto the surface and chilling for 2 hours.

PAIRING RECOMMENDED: Maple-Apple Topping

Chapter Twenty-seven

PUMPKIN PUDDING

YIELDS 6 SERVINGS

I adore pumpkin, whether it's roasted, stuffed, baked, sweet, or savoury, no matter how it's prepared. The idea for this meal occurred to me while I was celebrating Thanksgiving with my family and some friends a few years ago. I wanted to put my love of pumpkin into something spectacular, so I prepared a pudding that tasted exactly like pumpkin pie—warm spices, earthy pumpkin, just the right amount of sweetness—but instead of a crust, I spooned it into glasses. An instant classic was produced after a spoonful of whipped cream was added.

a third of a cup of half-and-half

1 34 gallon whole milk

3 beaten egg yolks

a third of a cup of cornstarch

1 unsweetened solid-pack pumpkin (15 oz.)

1 cup sugar, dark brown

1 teaspoon kosher salt

1/8 teaspoon nutmeg powder

1/8 teaspoon ginger powder

12 teaspoon cinnamon powder

1 teaspoon extract de vanille

1. In a medium saucepan, briskly whisk together all of the ingredients, except the vanilla extract, in a medium saucepan.

2. Cook, whisking continually, for 10 minutes over medium heat, until thickened. (It's done when you can raise the whisk from the pudding and see a faint shadow.)

3. Strain the pudding into a bowl through a fine-mesh sieve, squeezing the pudding through the sieve with a ladle (using a ladle here really helps separate the pumpkin solids from the silky pudding). Whisk in the vanilla extract.

4. Allow it cool for 10 minutes at room temperature before pressing a layer of plastic wrap onto the surface and chilling for 2 hours.

GRAHAM CRUMBS AND WHIPPED CREAM ARE SUGGESTED PAIRINGS

Chapter Twenty-eight

CHOCOLATE BROWNIES

MAKES 16 CUPS CRUMBS OR 16 BROWNIES

You already know I prefer vanilla, but these brownies, modified from The Barefoot Contessa Cookbook, are something I could eat again and over again. What more can I say about the rich chocolate flavour and smoky coffee undertones? Although these are intended to be crumbled as a topping for puddings, the recipe yields enough for you to munch on some whole.

melting 112 stick butter

12 ounces finely chopped bittersweet chocolate (70 percent cocoa)

1 ounce coarsely chopped unsweetened chocolate

sugar (34 cup)

two eggs

4 teaspoons espresso powder (instant)

1 tbsp extract de vanille

a third of a cup of all-purpose flour

2 teaspoons soda bicarbonate

1 tsp. salt (kosher)

1. Preheat the oven to 350 degrees Fahrenheit. Cooking spray a 9-by-9-inch baking sheet.

2. Melt the butter, 6 ounces bittersweet chocolate, and the unsweetened chocolate in a double boiler, stirring constantly, for 5–6 minutes. Remove the bowl from the heat and set aside to cool for 30 minutes.

3. Whisk together the sugar, eggs, espresso powder, and vanilla in a separate basin.

4. Whisk the egg mixture into the chocolate mixture until it is completely combined.

5. Combine the remaining bittersweet chocolate, flour, baking soda, and salt in a third basin. Fold the chocolate mixture using a spatula.

6. Pour the batter into the prepared pan and bake for 30–35 minutes, or until a toothpick inserted in the centre comes out clean.

7. Allow to cool to room temperature before crumbling and layering with your favourite pudding.

Chapter Twenty-nine

CHOCOLATE CHIPS COOKIES

COOKIES FOR 12 SANDWICHES OR 3 CUPS COOKIE CRUMBS

I've always had a thing for the iconic chocolate sandwich cookie, but not for the reasons you may expect. It's not the dark chocolate or even the filling that lingers after a bite, but the hauntingly slight sense of salt. I believe I've approximated the effect after a lot of trial and error. Kosher salt adds a familiar flavour that you won't be able to place in my rendition.

TO MAKE COOKIES:

10 teaspoons softened butter

12 cup of sugar

a quarter cup of light brown sugar

a single egg

12 teaspoon extract de vanille

3 tablespoons all-purpose flour plus 1 cup all-purpose flour

cocoa powder (1 cup)

2 tblsp. salt (kosher)

IN ORDER TO FILL:

1 softened stick of butter

1 cup room temperature vegetable shortening

2 CUP CONFECTIONERS' SUCTIONERS' SUCTIONERS'

vanilla extract (two teaspoons)

COOKIES TO MAKE:

1. Cream the butter, sugar, and brown sugar together in a stand mixer fitted with the paddle attachment for 1–2 minutes, or until fluffy.

2. Add the egg and vanilla extract and mix for another 1–2 minutes, stopping and scraping down the sides of the mixer as needed.

3. Combine flour and cocoa powder in a separate basin.

4. With the mixer turned off, add the flour-cocoa mixture to the bowl, then turn it on low speed and mix for 1–2 minutes, scraping down the sides of the bowl as needed.

5. Transfer dough to a clean work surface, flatten into a 4-inch-diameter disc, wrap in plastic wrap, and chill for 2 hours, or until firm. 30 minutes before usage, take the dough out of the refrigerator to soften it somewhat.

6. Preheat the oven to 350 degrees Fahrenheit.

7. Sprinkle the salt on two parchment-lined cookie sheets and set them aside.

8. On a lightly floured work surface, roll out the cookie dough to a thickness of 14 inches.

9. Cut out as many cookies as you can with a 4-inch round cookie cutter (you should end up with 24 cookies total). Transfer the cookies on the salted cookie sheet using an offset spatula. Because these cookies don't spread out much when baking, you can virtually stack them next to each other. Reroll remaining dough scraps into a ball, chilling slightly in the refrigerator if needed, and shape more cookies. Roll away—this dough is up to the task!

10. Bake the cookies for 15–20 minutes, or until they smell like thoroughly toasted chocolate.

11. Take the cookies out of the oven and allow them to cool completely on the baking sheet.

TO MAKE THE FILLING:

1. Cream butter and shortening in the bowl of a stand mixer fitted with the paddle attachment until smooth.

2. With the mixer turned off, pour confectioners' sugar into the mixing bowl. On medium-low speed, beat until completely combined, scraping down the sides of the bowl as needed.

3. Add the vanilla extract and beat on high speed for 3–4 minutes, or until super-creamy and fluffy.

COOKIES TO ASSEMBLE:

1. Fill a pastry bag or a ziplock bag with the filling and cut off one bottom corner.

2. Place half of the cookies salt-side down on a baking sheet and pipe 2 tablespoons filling into each, leaving a 12-inch border around the sides.

3. Place a second cookie on top of each, salt-side up, and gently press down so the filling spreads to the corners.

4. Set aside for 30 minutes to chill the cookies. Eat it plain or crumble it up and cover it with your favourite pudding.

MAKES 20 TWO-INCH COOKIES OR 5 CUPS CRUMBLES WITH GINGER CRUNCH

I may obsess over this pudding or that topping for months at a time, but these buttery squares are always fetish-worthy in my book. My mother was employed to prepare desserts for a New Zealand bakery, and she was given this recipe by Sue Boyer, a talented antipodean pastry chef. The crunchy cookie base, spicy taste, and luscious, velvety texture had everyone going crazy. They lend the ideal buttery zest to citrus puddings when finely crushed. You can also store them whole in the fridge or freezer and serve them cold—the chewy texture and subtle heat will keep you wanting more!

212 oz. softened butter, split

sugar (34 cup)

214 cup flour (all-purpose)

a total of 112 tablespoons baking powder

1 CUP CONFECTIONERS' SUCTIONERS' SUCTIONERS'

Lyle's Golden Syrup or light corn syrup, 3 teaspoons

312 teaspoons ginger powder

1. Preheat the oven to 350 degrees Fahrenheit. Cooking spray a 10-by-12-inch rimmed baking sheet, then top with parchment paper, spray again, and set aside.

2. In a normal mixer set with the paddle attachment, cream together 114 sticks of butter and the sugar for 3 minutes, or until fluffy. It will look that the mixture is dry; the longer you beat it, the better.

3. Add the flour and baking powder to the mixer while it is turned off. Blend on low speed to blend, then increase to medium and mix for 1–2 minutes, scraping down the sides of the bowl once.

4. Dump the dough onto the baking sheet that has been prepared. It won't appear to be enough dough at first, but trust me, it is. Make sure the dough is equally distributed throughout the pan and that it is as flat as possible. If desired, push the dough down with the bottom of a measuring cup or a glass.

5. Bake for 20 minutes, or until the dough is pale in the centre and the sides are just beginning to brown. (It's acceptable if the dough puffs up during baking!)

6. While the dough is baking, combine the remaining 114 sticks butter, confectioners' sugar, golden syrup, and ginger in a medium saucepan. Bring to a boil, then reduce to a low heat and continue to cook for 2 minutes, or until the syrup thickens and begins to peel away from the sides of the pan.

7. Remove the baking sheet from the oven and pour the syrup over the cookie slab right away. Make 20 two-inch squares out of the slab.

8. Allow it cool completely before eating or crumbling on top of your favourite pudding.

Chapter Thirty

GRAHAM CRACKERS

THIS RECIPE MAKES 24 GRAHAM CRACKERS

Graham crackers are a dessert with an identity crisis. They're not quite a cracker, and they're not quite cookie material, either. They began as a health-food item made using a specific sort of flour, but nowadays, most do not contain graham flour. I prefer to utilise the actual item for authenticity's sake—the real article should have noticeable deeper brown specks of wheat bran and germ. I roast the graham flour to provide depth, then combine it with two additional flours to create a perfect trio that balances tenderness and crispiness in every bite. The cookies are made slightly spicy by adding a pinch of black pepper.

12 cup graham flour (Bob's Red Mill is best)

1 cup flour (whole wheat)

a third of a cup of all-purpose flour

1 teaspoon kosher salt

12 tbsp baking soda

12 teaspoon cinnamon powder

14 teaspoon black pepper, freshly ground

2 teaspoons softened butter

2 tbsp. room temperature vegetable shortening

a third of a cup of light brown sugar

two eggs

14 cup of honey

vanilla extract (two teaspoons)

1. Preheat the oven to 350 degrees Fahrenheit.

2. On a parchment-lined rimmed baking sheet, spread graham flour evenly. Bake for 20 minutes, stirring after 10 minutes, or until flour darkens in colour (but not too much) and smells roasty-toasty. Allow to cool completely.

3. Combine graham flour, whole-wheat flour, all-purpose flour, salt, baking soda, cinnamon, and pepper in a large mixing basin and set aside.

4. In the bowl of a stand mixer fitted with the paddle attachment, beat the butter, shortening, brown sugar, and eggs on medium-high speed for 30 seconds, or until completely integrated.

5. Beat in the honey and vanilla for a further minute, or until smooth.

6. With the mixer on low speed, add half of the dry ingredients and beat for 1 minute, or until barely combined. Stop the mixer, scrape down the sides of the bowl, and add the remaining

dry ingredients. Return to medium-high speed and mix for another 30–60 seconds, or until just mixed, being careful not to overmix. (The dough will be quite tender.) Collect dough, wrap in plastic wrap, and refrigerate for at least 4 hours or overnight in the refrigerator while daydreaming about how delicious these graham crackers will be.

7. Roll out dough into a 14-inch-thick rectangle, about 10 x 15 inches, on parchment paper.

8. Cut dough into twenty-four 212-inch squares with a pizza cutter or a knife and ruler. Prick holes in each biscuit with a fork or pastry docker in any pattern you like.

9. Separate dough rectangles and place 12 inch apart on a parchment-lined cookie sheet (cookies will hardly spread).

10. Bake for 17–18 minutes, or until golden brown. Before serving, allow it cool to room temperature.

• MAKES 2 POUNDS OF CRUMBS

11 Graham Crackers or 5 2 12 by 5 inch store-bought graham cracker sheets

1 stick melted butter

a quarter cup of light brown sugar

1. Preheat the oven to 350 degrees Fahrenheit.

2. Place graham crackers in a food processor and pulse for 30 seconds, or until fine crumbs form.

3. Transfer the crumbs to a mixing dish and toss in the melted butter and brown sugar until the crumbs are coated.

4. Spread crumbs equally on a parchment-lined rimmed baking sheet and bake until toasted and aromatic, 12-14 minutes, stirring every 5 minutes.

5. Remove from the oven and set aside to cool completely. Your favourite pudding should be layered on top.

Chapter Thirty-one

VANILLA COOKIES

TURNS OUT APPROXIMATELY 412 DOZEN COOKIES

It took some trial and error to find the proper balance of tenderness and sharp edges, but now that I've nailed it, I can't get enough of these small round beauties. They're a terrific topping for any of our puddings, but I dare you to get that far without slipping one into a glass of milk on its own.

sugar (34 cup)

14 CUP CONFECTIONERS' SUCTIONERS' SUCTIONERS' SUCTIONERS

1 softened stick of butter

a quarter teaspoon of salt

two eggs

1 tablespoon milk (whole)

1 teaspoon extract de vanille

12 cup flour (all-purpose)

1 teaspoon powdered baking soda

1. Preheat the oven to 350 degrees Fahrenheit.

2. In the bowl of a stand mixer fitted with the paddle attachment, beat together the sugar, confectioners' sugar, butter, and salt on high speed for 3–4 minutes, scraping down the sides of the bowl as needed.

3. Reduce the speed to medium and add the eggs one at a time, beating well after each addition.

4. Beat in the milk and vanilla for 1 minute, or until fully combined.

5. Turn mixer off, add flour and baking powder, return to medium speed, and beat for 2–3 minutes, or until it looks like a thick spread. Refrigerate the dough for at least 30 minutes.

6. Drop batter by heaping teaspoonfuls onto two parchment-lined cookie sheets, about 1 inch apart (the batter dots may look small, but they spread out quite a bit when baking).

7. Bake for 15 minutes, changing cookie sheets after 7 minutes, until golden brown along the edges and pale in the centre. On a cookie sheet, cool thoroughly.

Chapter Thirty-two

DULCE DE LECHE PUDDING

MAKES 1-1\2 CUPS

This recipe was initially intended for use in my Dulce de Leche Pudding, but it was far too excellent to be relegated to a single recipe. So here it is, all golden and ready to be spooned upon your favourite pudding (or turned into national currency). Making dulce de leche straight in the can is a long-standing Latin custom; the method is easy, and the result is seductive. Opening the can after cooking is a revelation, as the condensed milk has thickened and darkened to the most beautiful golden tint you've ever seen.

1 can sweetened condensed milk, 14 oz

1. In a small saucepan, pour an unopened 14-ounce can of sweetened condensed milk. Fill the saucepan with water until it reaches 34 percent of the way up the can's edges.

2. Over high heat, bring the pot to a boil, then reduce to a hard simmer. Allow to simmer for at least 3 hours and up to 5 hours,

rotating the can every 30 minutes and adding extra water when the level on the edges of the can reduces to halfway.

3. Remove can from water with a jar lifter, tongs, or heatproof oven mitt and set aside to cool until easy to handle, about 30 minutes. Warm or at room temperature is fine.

• YIELDS 112 CUPS

The combination of berries and wine creates a nearly Port-like syrup in this compote, and the unexpected addition of lime adds a zingy edge that makes it perfect as a topper for Hevra's Lemon Obsession Pudding, Happens-to-Be-Vegan Coconut Pudding, or Key Lime Pudding.

12 cup blackberries (distributed)

14 cup red wine, dry and fruity

14 cup of sugar

lime juice (two teaspoons)

34 cup blackberries, wine, sugar, and lime juice in a small pot Bring to a boil, then remove from the heat, toss in the remaining blackberries, and set aside to cool.

• THIS RECIPE MAKES 212 CUPS

Use Montmorency cherries for this tart-sweet compote; they're a delightful sour kind that gives the end result a puckery sweetness. Though I prefer this compote on Vanilla Pudding, it's also delicious on morning porridge, spooned onto angel food cake, or atop Greek yoghurt.

12 cup red wine, dry and fruity

12 cup of sugar

2 cups dried sweetened pitted cherries

1. In a small saucepan, bring the wine, 34 cup water, and sugar to a boil.

2. Remove from heat, add cherries, and set aside for 5 minutes in the hot liquid. Compote can be served warm or cold, and it can be kept in the refrigerator for up to a week in an airtight container or ziplock bag.

• THIS RECIPE SERVES 2 CUPS

This was created to accompany my Christmas Parfait, but it would also be delicious mixed with a bowl of Greek yoghurt or used as a condiment for a holiday dinner. This compote is distinguished from others I've tried by the addition of fresh ginger.

12 oz. bag of fresh cranberries

sugar (34 cup)

12 CUP OLIVE JUICE

12 orange zest

1 tablespoon ginger, finely grated

In a medium saucepan, bring the cranberries, 34 cup water, sugar, orange juice, and zest to a boil. Reduce heat to low and cook for 15–20 minutes, or until cranberries have broken up and the sauce has thickened. During the last minute of cooking, add the ginger. Cool. Compote can be kept in the refrigerator for up to a week in an airtight container or ziplock bag.

• THIS RECIPE SERVES 3 CUPS

Peach Melba was first introduced to me in high school, after a naive attempt at low-fat cooking. (Wait a minute, what was I thinking?) This light and delightful combination of fresh fruit and sugar, prepared gently, was created by renowned chef Auguste Escoffier in honour of Australian opera star Nellie Melba.

14 cup of sugar

3 cups peeled, pitted, and diced ripe peaches or two 10-ounce packages thawed frozen sliced peaches

a third of a cup of raspberries

Bring sugar and 14 cup water to a boil in a medium pot. Simmer for 3 minutes, or until peaches are slightly softened. Remove the pan from the heat and add the berries. Allow to cool to room temperature before chilling in the refrigerator. Compote can be kept in the refrigerator for up to a week in an airtight container or ziplock bag.

• THIS RECIPE SERVES 2 CUPS

This light, maple-laced topping is best when made with Grade B maple syrup, which is often darker and more liquidy than Grade A syrup and loaded with overtones of smoke and wood—almost like a fine bourbon—and is great as part of our Breakfast of Champions Parfait.

14 cup melted butter

2 large, crisp apples (about 1 pound total), peeled, cored, and diced

a quarter teaspoon of cinnamon

12 CUP MAPLE SUGAR

a quarter teaspoon of salt

1. Melt butter in a small saucepan over medium heat for 1–2 minutes, or until brown and flecked with tiny toasted bits.

2. Add the apples and cinnamon and cook for 5 minutes, or until the apples are slightly softened.

3. Add the maple syrup and salt, bring to a boil, then reduce heat to low and continue to cook for another 2 minutes. Remove the pan from the heat and allow it cool to room temperature. Warm or at room temperature is fine. For up to a week, put the topping in an airtight container or ziplock bag in the refrigerator.

• THIS RECIPE SERVES 2 CUPS

The richness of the pudding is perfectly balanced by unsweetened whipped cream. The unadulterated cream, whipped into a pillowy cloud, cuts the sweetness of the pudding and adds a light, airy touch.

1 cup heavy cream, cold

Whip cream in the bowl of a stand mixer fitted with the whisk attachment on high speed for 1–2 minutes, or until soft peaks form.

• SERVES 214 CUPS

Take whipped cream, for example. Pour in the caramel sauce. Whip a little more. Enjoy—I mean, obsess about it. As we do in the shop, we're completely obsessed. If I could, I'd use this stuff to paint the walls! The caramel gives the cream more substance without taking away from its volume, resulting in golden clouds. You'll want to float away with a bowlful, trust me.

1 cup heavy cream, cold

2/3 cup chilled salted caramel sauce

1. Whip cream in the bowl of a stand mixer fitted with the whisk attachment on high speed for 1–2 minutes, or until soft peaks form.

2. Whip in the Salted Caramel Sauce for a further 2 minutes, or until soft peaks appear.

CPSIA information can be obtained
at www.ICGtesting.com
Printed in the USA
LVHW061835130722
723448LV00014B/178

9 781804 768372